# SCIATICA NERVE PAIN

### Symptoms, Tests, and Treatment for Lumbar Radiculopathy

## Nicholas Gallo, PT, DPT

# DISCLAIMER

---

The contents of this book are based on my personal experiences as a Board Certified Physical Therapist and are for informational purposes only. This book does not constitute medical advice; the content of this book is not intended to be a substitute for professional medical advice, diagnosis, or treatment. Always seek the advice of a physician or other qualified health provider with any questions you may have regarding a medical condition. Never disregard professional medical advice or delay in seeking it because of something you have read on this website. Reliance on any information provided by this book is solely at your own risk.

# TABLE OF CONTENTS

———

# INTRODUCTION

---

Sciatica nerve pain can be debilitating and very frustrating. It can become life-changing, and the pain and discomfort can make people feel helpless. The available treatments range from conservative management to surgical management. In my experience, a person with sciatica nerve pain can be treated conservatively with physical therapy exercises and achieve great outcomes. Don't just take my word for it, though; let me cite some research for you. In a study by Boote et al., they cited research stating that "surgery generates improved outcomes in the short term, but at 1 year, outcomes are very similar in both physiotherapy and surgical groups." What is the significance of this, you ask? It means that, although surgical options may provide great short-term relief, similar (if not the same) results can be achieved without surgery. This is a pretty significant finding because some patients think that surgery is their only option for relief.

Typically, sciatica nerve pain can be treated via stretching, strengthening, and sciatic nerve mobilizations. What I find most often is that people do not know which things to perform and/or how to perform them correctly. Therefore, for each treatment I talk about, I will go into detail on how to perform them correctly and why it works. I will also go into detail on specific positions and postures to avoid so that you can decrease the amount of pain you are in. Finally, I will include specific sleeping positions and other clinically proven methods that can help relieve this pain experienced by so many people. By using this step-by-step systematic approach, it is my goal that you begin to experience relief and get back to your normal routine.

Therefore, in this publication I will outline effective conservative treatment options for sciatica nerve pain that are proven in the research community. I have personally applied these treatment options when working with individuals with this condition in my experience as a board-certified doctor of physical therapy. I have personally seen the benefits of these methods, and I want to make them more well known amongst people suffering from this condition.

I also have a variety of free educational videos showing a variety of different treatments and diagnoses on my YouTube channel *Physical Therapy 101*. This channel was started to provide free, to-the-point exercises to patients and practitioners. This channel is continuously being updated and provides a slew of information spanning several diagnoses including sciatica, so please subscribe if you are interested. Supplemental information can be found on my website www.physicaltherapy101.net. If you would also like to join my email list, send me an email at nickgallodpt@gmail.com. I will email you directly with new publications and videos I publish as soon as they come out so that you have exclusive access to them.

# WHAT IS SCIATICA?

First off, let's go over what sciatica is. The term "sciatica" is defined as "pain along the course of the sciatic nerve or its branches." You may be asking yourself, "Now, what is the sciatic nerve?" The sciatic nerve is a large nerve that begins in the lower back and extends down the buttock and lower limb. Therefore, sciatica nerve pain is characterized by pain that originates in the lower back and extends down the lower limb along the nerve distribution.

The sciatic nerve is massive. During cadaver lab in graduate school we dissected this area so that we could visualize it. It is significant to see its size and location because of where it is found anatomically. It passes directly under a muscle known as the piriformis. I'll go into further detail later about why this muscle is important, but know that this muscle can play a major role in why a person is feeling their symptoms.

As the sciatic nerve passes through this muscle, it extends down the rest of the lower extremity into several branches and provides innervation to the rest of the leg. I won't go into any more boring anatomy details. However, I am explaining this because this is why people with sciatica flare-ups may feel pain extending down their lower extremity.

# WHERE IS SCIATICA
# PAIN COMMONLY FELT?

---

Building more on this point, I want to go into detail on where specifically a person may feel sciatica pain. Commonly, patients experience sciatica nerve pain in their gluteal region and it can move down the back of their thigh. Due to the extensions of the nerve further down the leg, it is not abnormal to also feel pain and discomfort extending into the lower leg and/or foot. When I say "pain" or "discomfort," I want you to know this can vary depending on the individual. I have heard all of the following descriptions for a person's sciatica: dull ache, sharp pain, burning sensations, numbness, tingling, and electric shock pain. Just know that if you are feeling one of those types of pains and it is following the nerve pathway, this is consistent with sciatica.

Sciatica nerve pain may also result in the decreased power, sensation, and reflexes in these areas. Sometimes people will feel weakness in their lower limb and say that one side feels weaker than the other. The best way to confirm these symptoms is by seeing a healthcare practitioner and having a proper evaluation.

# WHAT CAUSES SCIATICA?

There are a few things that can lead to sciatica nerve pain. Common causes include: herniated disc, spinal stenosis, and entrapment of the sciatic nerve. All three of these may result in compression and/or irritation of the sciatic nerve and lead to the symptoms I listed before. It is important to know that the sciatic nerve in this case is considered the "victim," and the underlying condition causing the irritation is known as the "culprit." I like to typically outline to patients what is causing their discomfort and which structures are affected. In this case, the structure being affected is the sciatic nerve, and the underlying condition is something causing the irritation. Other possible causes, although rare, include tumors and other abnormal growths. Therefore, it is imperative to get these rarities ruled out before proceeding with a treatment plan.

Now, I want to be clear at this point: just because an MRI shows that you have a spine abnormality, it does NOT necessarily mean that you are symptomatic. Brinjikji et al. performed a systematic review where they looked at MRIs for over 3,000 people who did not experience lower back symptoms. What they found was that approximately 30% of those 20 years of age had some type of disc-related pathology, and this number increased with age. Also, approximately 37% of those 20 years of age also had disc degeneration in their MRI results. You may ask yourself, "Now, why are they not symptomatic with these findings?"

That is because imaging results do not always dictate how a person presents. I have seen this time and again while treating individuals over the years. Just because the imaging shows a disc pathology, this absolutely does not mean that you are doomed.

When it comes to people who are symptomatic with sciatica nerve pain, however, approximately 90% of cases are due to herniated disc with compression on a nerve root. This nerve root compression is what causes those shooting pains going down a person's lower extremity. The location of a person's symptoms usually depends on the nerve root that is affected. I will elaborate on a herniated disc later, but it is important to know that according to the research at hand, sciatica is most commonly associated with having a herniated disc.

# RISK FACTORS FOR SCIATICA

There have been some studies about risk factors for sciatica in order to determine whether there are factors that predispose people to sciatica symptoms. I like to include these when I evaluate a new patient because they may play a pivotal role in a person's reduction of symptoms. First off, one risk factor that has been examined extensively is smoking. Although the specific mechanism on how smoking increases sciatica pain is not specifically known, smoking has been shown to decrease nutrition to the disc in the spine. Smoking has also been shown to increase disc inflammation and prevent healing of these areas. Therefore, if someone is a smoker and they are experiencing very bad pain, I suggest that they try to quit.

Another big risk factor for sciatica is being overweight/obese. One proposed mechanism of how this occurs is that obesity has been shown to delay the healing process in these areas. Carrying around excess weight also places more strain on the spine and other structures, which can lead to the exacerbation of sciatica symptoms. Body weight is a sensitive topic; however, I always tell a person that fits these criteria that they are outside of their ideal weight range because this is another characteristic they can improve on. I won't go into the different methods of weight loss, but typically I suggest that people begin with lower-impact exercise such as walking, so that they can start getting more active.

This is not a risk factor, but it is worth mentioning that sciatica can also be experienced during pregnancy. Although not officially determined, some mechanisms have been proposed to try and explain this. First off, weight gain during the pregnancy process can place additional strain on a person's spine and cause irritation. Also, there are significant hormonal changes that occur during pregnancy, which are also believed to play a role in causing sciatica. If this is the case, I always make sure the patient has had an extensive medical examination by their healthcare practitioners before we begin treatment.

# SCIATICA EMERGENCIES

Before I begin discussing tests and exercises, I want to make sure you know when your symptoms are consistent with a medical emergency. These symptoms should not be taken lightly. As soon as you experience them, you should seek medical attention right away. If you ignore them, you may do harm to yourself that is irreparable.

The first question I always ask people is, "Are you having any bowel or bladder incontinence?" By this I mean whether they are having any issues controlling their bowel and bladder function. This is significant because it is a primary symptom of a condition known as cauda equina syndrome. This syndrome is essentially damage to the bundle of nerves below the spinal cord, also known as the cauda equina. Although this is a rare condition, it does happen and it requires immediate medical attention. Failure to seek help may result in the permanent loss of bowel and bladder control and/or paralysis of the lower limbs.

The next question I ask people is, "Are your symptoms getting significantly worse?" The symptoms that I am most concerned about are whether they are losing significant motor function of the affected area. If you are progressively losing strength and feeling as if the affected limb is getting substantially worse, this is also a medical emergency. It can mean that the sciatic nerve is substantially damaged and/or the nerves involved are continually getting compressed. Worsening symptoms in the leg may also be the result of cauda equina syndrome. Therefore, this should be brought to the attention of a medical professional right away.

Finally, there are some additional conditions. If you meet them, it is absolutely necessary to get examined by a medical professional first to rule out any of these pathologies. These conditions are known as red flags and are things that I ask about when I evaluate any new patient. Here is a list of some conditions and what they can potentially mean:

- Recent major trauma could indicate a fracture.
- Medical history of cancer could indicate a tumor.
- Fever, chills, and/or night sweats could indicate an infection or tumor.
- Night pain could indicate an infection or tumor.
- Compromised immune system could indicate an infection.

This is just a brief list of potential symptoms and causes of those symptoms other than sciatica. Therefore, if a patient has any of these symptoms above, I typically suggest that they follow up with their primary care doctor to rule out any serious underlying condition.

# SCIATIC NERVE TESTS

Now that you have some background information on sciatica and have ruled out any serious underlying pathology, I want to go over some great tests that can be done to determine if what a person is experiencing is sciatica nerve pain. You may have already undergone these tests if you've seen your healthcare provider or you may have seen these somewhere on the internet. These tests are specifically designed to evaluate the neural tissues of the spinal cord. If they have a tendency to reproduce your discomfort, then chances are you are experiencing sciatica.

## The Slump Test

This test is very accurate in determining whether there is some nerve involvement in a patient's pain. It is also a very accurate and quick assessment, so it is frequently used in the clinical setting.

1. To begin, the patient will sit up straight in a chair or on the edge of their bed with their head in a neutral position.

2. Next, they allow themselves to slump like they are slouching into bad posture, allowing their shoulders to round while maintaining their head in neutral.

3. If their symptoms are not reproduced, they bend their head forward and allow their chin to touch their chest. Next, they begin to straighten one of

their legs and have their toes pointed forward in an ankle motion known as plantarflexion.

4. To further advance this test, as they straighten their leg, they then point their toes back at themselves in an ankle motion known as dorsiflexion.

5. If negative, perform the same steps on the other leg.

This slump test may reproduce your symptoms and you might be asking yourself, "Why does this happen?" When you are fully slumped forward, you allow your spine to bend forward. This motion is known as flexion. When you combine this position with straightening out your lower extremity, you tense your neural tissues. If something such as a disc herniation is compressing a nerve tissue or impinging on it, you will experience pain and tightness.

**Straight Leg Raise Test**

Another test that can be used in combination with the slump test is known as the straight leg raise test. This test was the first test to look at neural tissue and is still used today due to its accuracy.

1. To begin, lay down on your back.

2. One leg is raised passively by the healthcare provider until subjective reports of pain or stretching are felt in the leg.

3. To further advance the test, the toes are bent back towards the patient in the ankle dorsiflexion position.
4. This test is repeated on the other side and compared.

The straight leg raise test may reproduce your symptoms due to placing tension on the sciatic nerve and neural structures. It is not uncommon to experience tightness in the back of your thigh during this test. A positive result is if this amplifies your sciatica nerve pain.

# POSTURE CORRECTIONS

---

Posture is a massive subject and I have written another publication exclusively on this subject. When dealing with sciatica, however, make no exception: YOUR POSTURE IS SIGNIFICANT. Therefore, I want to go over specific postures and corrections you should make when managing your symptoms. If you want to learn in full detail how to modify your desk and help achieve this throughout the work day, my publication "Posture Pain: Key Strategies to Stay Pain-Free at Your Desk and in Life" is right up your alley.

First and foremost, when you sit for long periods of time, this leads to compression on your sciatic nerve. I tell people it's like falling asleep on your arm: when you wake up eventually, you get that numbness and tingling sensation. When you sit, the same thing can happen to your sciatic nerve, especially if it is already inflamed or irritated. Therefore, I encourage people to get up and walk around when their sciatica nerve pain starts to worsen.

When you are sitting, it is also important that you don't lean to one side or the other. You want to make sure you are sitting evenly on both of your glutes. Shifting your weight to one side or the other is a bad compensatory mechanism that people do naturally, but it can lead to more complications down the line. Therefore, it's important that you be mindful of how you are sitting. If you need some help with this, try sitting in front of a mirror so you can see how you are sitting subconsciously.

When sitting, be very mindful of whether you are slouching forward or not. One of the tests I went over earlier for sciatica was the slump test. If that test is positive, you already know that slumping forward reproduces your pain. Even if you were not symptomatic for this test, I advise you to avoid this posture. Sitting in a posture that allows your head to fall forward and your shoulders to round places strain on your lower back and can increase pain if you are already experiencing it. Therefore, try to sit up straight and avoid these bad habits.

# SLEEPING POSITIONS

---

One aspect of daily life that I believe is overlooked in the recovery process is how people sleep. If you think about it, we put ourselves in these positions for long periods of time so that we can fall asleep. I realize that we do not maintain these positions the entire time we are asleep and some people move. It is important, however, to be mindful of the correct ways to sleep when dealing with sciatica so that you are not doing more harm than good.

## Sleeping on Your Back

A position that I have found effective for many people who are experiencing sciatica is sleeping on their back with their knees elevated. You may have already discovered this, but try lying on your back with your knees bent and feet flat. Does this position feel better than having your legs flat? If you feel like this position will be beneficial for you, it is easy to try and maintain this position for a while when you try to go to sleep. Usually, what I suggest is that a patient gets into this position and then places pillows underneath their knees so that they can relax and maintain this sleeping position. You can also buy certain items such as bolsters to go under the knees. Many clinics (mine included) have those on offer. Nevertheless, bolsters are not completely necessary to purchase. I have found that using pillows can be just as effective.

Typically, people find this position to be relieving for their sciatica because by having your knees elevated, you place less pressure on the discs and nerve roots. The best way to start with this position is by having your buttocks and feet maintain contact with your sleeping surface. If you want to try and raise the height of your knees, I suggest to do that slowly. Also, if it does not work right away, try it for a few more days and modify accordingly.

## Sleeping on Your Side

If you are a side sleeper, this can be frustrating because symptoms may increase as the night goes on. As we sleep on our side, our hips and spine may get out of alignment and can increase sciatica symptoms. Therefore, I like to suggest to people that they place a pillow between their knees when lying on their side. I want you to try this position. Do things begin to feel more comfortable? Placing a pillow between your knees while lying on your side allows the hips, spine, and pelvis to maintain more of a neutral alignment. A normal pillow can work for this, but I have also had patients tell me that a body pillow was really effective when side sleeping. Therefore, experiment and find which method is the best for you.

Another thing I suggest to people is that they try their best not to sleep on the side where they experience sciatica pain. I have them avoid this because sleeping on the affected side places additional pressure on the already irritated nerve. I know that people commonly move in their sleep and shift positions, which can make this difficult. What I like to suggest to people is to place a pillow or raised surface on the side where they experience sciatica pain. As the person rolls to that side in their sleep, this raised surface can prevent them from lying completely flat.

## Sleeping on Your Stomach

Many people like to sleep on their stomachs. I am not a big fan of this position. First off, this tends to flatten the natural curve of the spine, which is not recommended. It also allows the spine to go into a motion known as hyperextension and can place excess strain on the spine. Finally, since people typically turn their head to one side or the other, this can lead to neck strains and pains when repeated. Therefore, I usually suggest that people try to sleep on their unaffected side and/or their back as I described before.

If you find yourself only comfortable on your stomach, then there is a modification that I suggest people make. Since lying on your stomach causes the spine to lose its natural curvature, I suggest that people place a pillow underneath their abdomen. This allows a person's spine to maintain more of a natural curvature compared to having nothing beneath it. Also, a softer mattress tends to allow the lower back to move into more of a hyperextension compared to a firmer mattress. Therefore, you may need to look at a specific type of mattress, as I will discuss next.

# SLEEPING SURFACE

———

This is a highly variable topic among people that are having sciatica pain. I have heard everything from sleeping on the floor, sleeping in a recliner, and sleeping on all types of different mattresses. One is not necessarily better than the other because every person is unique. What I can suggest is that you try out several and see how you feel in the morning. When people initially come to me, I have them rate their pain on a scale of 1 to 10, with 1 being the lowest and 10 being the highest. I want you to do the same with regards to your sleeping surface. If you feel improvement, take note and try to modify further so that you are completely comfortable and can sleep well the entire night.

I also commonly get questions regarding mattress types. Just like sleeping positions and sleeping surfaces, this is very subjective. I have people that swear by certain mattress types and others that I cannot give a specific recommendation on this. What I can suggest is that there are so many out there that if you are looking to purchase a new one, go try out as many as you can and make a decision. One option that can provide many possibilities are the mattresses of which you can adjust the firmness. I do not personally have a lot of experience with these and I have read that they can be very expensive, but varying the firmness can be very effective for people. This makes sense in that you can give yourself a custom setting that you can continually adjust until it is perfect for your body.

# SCIATICA EXERCISES

---

I will list some great sciatica stretches and strengthening exercises that I have found to be effective when treating this condition. You can find all the ones I mention in a video on my YouTube channel titled "Exercises to Help with Sciatica During Pregnancy." This video was recorded for a colleague's wife because she was experiencing sciatica pain during pregnancy, but they are effective exercises that can work for anybody in this condition. (Note: the video also features other exercises and variations that you are free to try. I will only talk about the ones that have worked best in my experience.)

## Gluteal Stretches

One thing that is important when dealing with sciatica nerve pain is that you keep the tissues surrounding the sciatic nerve stretched and limber. It is important to remember that, when doing these stretches, you may start to feel some sciatica nerve pain. This is normal; however, you do not want to overstretch these tissues because overstretching can lead to more intense flare-ups of the nerve. Therefore, when you are stretching, you should stretch to the point RIGHT BEFORE you start to experience pain. Always let your symptoms be the judge of how far to stretch, as you do not want them to make you feel worse.

**Single Knee to Chest Stretch**

This stretch is performed just like the name suggests: you literally pull one knee to your chest. However, there are a few modifications that are important to try and prevent this from causing additional pain.

1. Lie on your back with both of your knees bent and feet resting flat on the floor.
2. In order to stretch the right side, cup your hands behind your right thigh and pull your knee gently to your chest.
3. If this is too intense or you have trouble grabbing behind your thigh, you can grab towards your leg where the shin meets your knee.
4. If this is also too difficult, you can place a strap behind your right thigh and pull the leg into position using the strap.
5. Perform 3-4 repetitions and hold for 20-30 seconds.
6. Once you have stretched your right side, perform this exercise on the left.

**Piriformis Stretch**

The piriformis is a muscle located on the pelvis that can play a major role in sciatica nerve pain. What's significant is its location with regards to the sciatic nerve. If the piriformis muscle is tight or goes into spasm, it can compress on the sciatic nerve and cause pain. In order to prevent this, it is important to keep the muscle stretched.

## Seated Piriformis Stretch

1. Begin by sitting in a sturdy chair.
2. To begin stretching the right side, cross your legs so that your right ankle is resting on the top of your left thigh.
3. To further intensify this stretch, try to push down your right knee so that your knee is parallel with the floor, creating a "Figure 4" position.
4. You can advance this stretch even further by maintaining an upright seated position and by leaning forward.
5. You should feel this stretch in your right hip and glute area.
6. Perform 3-4 repetitions and hold for 20-30 seconds.
7. Once you have stretched your right side, perform it on the left.

I like showing people this stretch in the seated position because they can do it everywhere, especially if they are at work and begin to feel pain.

## Supine Piriformis Stretch

The piriformis stretch can also be performed when lying down supine, and I encourage you to do this version as well. If lying on the floor is uncomfortable, you can perform it in bed.

1. Begin by lying on your back with both of your knees bent and feet flat on the floor.
2. To stretch your right side, cross your legs so that your right ankle is resting on the top of your left

thigh, creating that same "Figure 4" position as before.

3. Using your hands, pull your left thigh towards your chest while your right ankle remains on your left thigh.

4. If this is difficult, you can wrap a strap around your left thigh and pull on the strap with your hands.

5. Pull until you feel a stretch in your right hip and glute area.

6. Perform 3-4 repetitions and hold for 20-30 seconds.

7. Once you have stretched your right side, perform it on the left.

In the supine position, this exercise can be performed quickly in bed. I like to add it as the next progression to the seated exercise because this one can be more intense than that one. Therefore, I suggest trying the seated version first and then this one after the seated version becomes too easy.

# GLUTEAL STRENGTH

_____

We have gone over stretching the tissues surrounding the sciatic nerve. However, it is very important that the muscles surrounding it are strong too. There are three different types of gluteal muscles: gluteus maximus, gluteus minimus, and gluteus medius. They all play a major role in the stabilization of a person's pelvis and hip movements. If they are weak, a person will begin to compensate and have exacerbation of their pain. Therefore, I will go over a few of the gluteal strengthening exercises that I commonly prescribe to patients.

**Supine Bridges**

The bridge exercise is very beneficial when rehabilitating sciatica. It is an easy-to-do, low-impact exercise that really isolates the gluteal muscles. It can also be done without any equipment and be advanced fairly easily.

1. Start by lying on your back with your hands by your side and feet flat on the floor.
2. Tighten your core and buttock muscles.
3. Raise your bottom up until you create a straight line going from your shoulders to your knees.
4. Slowly allow your bottom to come back down.
5. Work up to 3 sets of 10 repetitions.

This exercise is simultaneously working your core, lower back, and gluteal muscles. Initially, this exercise may seem tough, but over time you will notice that it becomes easier. When this happens, it is important to advance the exercise to make it more difficult. One great way to do this is, instead of performing the bridge exercise with two feet, perform it with one foot. This is much more difficult than it sounds, and it is a great way to advance the exercise. If it is initially too hard, try doing the bridge exercise with both feet and then raising one while maintaining your hips at the same height. If you notice that your hips begin to fall back to the surface, then you have identified that you need to work on additional gluteal weakness.

**The Side-Lying Clamshell**

This exercise is most often prescribed because it allows strengthening of the gluteal muscles in a different plane of movement. It is also very low-impact; however, it will isolate the gluteus medius muscle effectively, which is important in the rehabilitation process for sciatica.

1. Start by lying on your side with the hip that you want to strengthen facing up.
2. Make sure your legs are stacked on top of each other and your knees are bent.
3. During the exercise, it's important to make sure your core is tight and engaged.
4. While keeping your feet touching, raise your top knee as high as you can without allowing your hips to rotate. If this is difficult for you, lie on your side with your back touching a wall to prevent movement.

5. Pause at the top and return to the starting position under control. Work up to 30 repetitions.
6. Repeat on the other side.
7. When it becomes too easy, add a resistance band around your thighs to make it harder.

I love this exercise because the gluteus medius muscle is so important for the rehabilitation of a patient with sciatica and lower back pain. Most commonly, as I mentioned above, people rotate their hips and the exercise will be ineffective. That is why it is of the utmost importance to make sure that you do not make that mistake.

## Sciatic Nerve Mobilization

Now that the surrounding tissues are stretched, it's important to perform some dynamic exercises that allow the sciatic nerve to be mobilized. Jeong et al. determined that, "Application of mobilization techniques for the sciatic nerves may promote healing of the soft tissues by stimulating the functions of the nervous system to improve nervous system adaptability and decrease sensitivity, helping to alleviate the symptoms." The group that experienced the most relief in this study performed these mobilization techniques in addition to other therapy exercises for lumbar stabilization. Therefore, I like to include these in my treatment plan along with some other treatments I will go over shortly.

It is important for you to realize that you can absolutely overstretch and cause additional pain with these exercises. That is why I always tell people to perform them right before they begin to feel pain and discomfort. The tissues being stretched and mobilized during these exercises are very sensitive, and flaring them up more is not the goal here. You also do not want to do more than 10 repetitions per day due to the sensitive nature of these exercises. I have recorded them in a video on my YouTube channel titled, "Sciatic Nerve Glides – Sciatic Nerve Entrapment Sciatica Pain Relief."

## Seated Sciatic Nerve Glides

A sciatic nerve glide is a technique used to help mobilize the sciatic nerve. What makes nerve glides different is that the nerve is mobilized via dynamic stretching. The first one I want to go over is the seated sciatic nerve glide because it can be done pretty much anywhere and at any time. This nerve glide may seem familiar to you because it is exactly the same position as the slump test I reviewed earlier. If you feel sciatica on one side of your body, perform this exercise on that side. However, I encourage people to do it on both sides because it will help keep you symmetrical.

1. To begin, sit up straight on a chair or on the edge of your bed with your head in a neutral position.
2. Next, straighten your leg with your toes pointed forward. If you are already feeling a reproduction of your symptoms, straighten your leg right before you begin to feel your symptoms and then allow your leg to bend again to the starting position.

3. To increase the intensity, straighten your leg and bend your toes back towards you.
4. If you would like to intensify this mobilization even further, allow your shoulders and head to slouch forward and repeat the previous step.
5. It is important to remember to not overstretch during this exercise.

**Supine Sciatic Nerve Glides**

The same mobilization technique can be done while lying supine. Like before, if you are not comfortable doing this on the floor, you can do it while lying in bed.

1. To begin, lie on your back with both knees bent.
2. Pull the affected thigh towards you until it is perpendicular to the ceiling.
3. In this position, allow your leg to straighten, with the toes pointing towards the ceiling. If you are already feeling a reproduction of your symptoms, straighten your leg right before you begin to feel your symptoms and then allow your leg to bend again to the starting position.
4. To increase the intensity, straighten your leg and bend your toes back towards you.
5. If you would like to intensify this mobilization even further, lift your head to your chest and repeat the prior steps.
6. Once again, DO NOT overstretch.

# HEAT OR ICE?

When I am treating people for sciatica nerve pain, I commonly get asked which is better: heat or ice? Everybody is so different that a "one-size-fits-all" approach does not always work, but I will explain what I was taught in school. Typically, if you want to reduce inflammation, ice should be used. This is best applied during the acute phase of an injury, which spans 3-7 days. After this inflammatory period, it is suggested that you start to use heat to enhance blood flow to the area and to promote healing. Heat and ice should be applied for approximately 15-20 minutes and can be performed multiple times per day as needed. These are good guidelines for the most part, but I would like to include some specifics that I have learned in my clinical experience.

First off, I sometimes include heat before a patient starts stretching and/or doing activities so that the tissues can loosen up. This helps decrease people's stiffness and allows muscles to stretch more easily. Heat also tends to allow tight muscles around the sciatic nerve to relax, thus decreasing compression on it. I usually do this if someone has been dealing with this injury for a long time and it is considered a chronic injury. After a person has completed their treatment session, if they have increased sciatica symptoms, I will provide them with ice to try and calm the sciatic nerve back down. This tends to decrease inflammation around the nerve, and it may numb the pain. This is not the same for every person, however, so I suggest that you start with this method and then play around with what works best for you.

There are a few important things to avoid if you are using these methods for pain relief.

First off, always use a towel or some sort of barrier between the ice or heat and your skin. I have seen people burn themselves and nearly get frostbite by avoiding this rule, which is completely avoidable! Also, try not to fall asleep when using these methods because ideally, they should be used for 15-20 minutes at a time. If you fall asleep, you may also damage your skin. One thing I really want to suggest is that you set an alarm to time yourself just in case you fall asleep. Also DO NOT stretch directly after applying ice therapy because this temporarily decreases the pliability of muscles.

# BONUS SECTION: LET'S TALK ABOUT DISC HERNIATIONS

---

Since I mentioned earlier that a herniated disc is fairly common and leads to sciatica nerve pain, I would like to talk about this subject. It can play a major role in the reduction of your symptoms. Intervertebral discs, also commonly referred to as just "discs," are located between our vertebrae. The disc provides a cushion between our vertebrae for compressive loads. If the disc is loaded too much or incorrectly, the material located inside may start to push on a nerve, which can lead to sciatica. Specifically, as I mentioned before, research has shown that 90% of sciatica cases are due to a disc herniation. Therefore, if we want to reduce sciatica symptoms, we also need to look at treating the disc directly.

## How Do Herniated Discs Happen?

Typically, people herniate a disc when they are putting a compressive load on the spine during flexion. You may have experienced this when you bend forward to pick something up and start to feel pain in the lower back. The pain may have occurred immediately or gradually, over time. The mechanism of injury is typically the same: bending forward places the compression on the front of the disc, and it will typically herniate backwards. The disc may also herniate to the side and cause compression on spinal nerves, which leads to the sciatica pain.

The combination of bending and lifting will increase your chances of disc herniation. However, when you also include twisting, then you increase your chances even further. In school we learned to "avoid BLTs (bending, lifting, twisting)." When you combine bending, lifting, and twisting, you greatly load the disc, which can further increase your chances of disc herniation. Therefore, if you do not have a disc herniation, then I suggest that you try to avoid these positions to prevent injury. If you already have some type of herniation, avoid doing this as well to prevent the further progression of herniation.

### Lifting Correctly From Floor

Since lifting something in a suboptimal position can lead to a disc herniation, I want to go into some details on proper lifting techniques. A lot of times people prevent any movement in their ankles and knees and try to lift with their lower back by bending over and rounding their spine. This places a lot of strain and motion on the spinal column and can lead to injury, more specifically a disc herniation. One way to lift something off of the floor properly is by bending the knees instead of the lower back. This causes more motion to be done at the hips, knees, and ankles instead of placing the strain on the lower back. You might have heard, "Lift with your legs," which is essentially the squatting position I am referring to here. Everybody's anatomy is different, so I suggest you play around and determine which squatting position works best for you.

Another way to properly lift something off of the floor is known as the "golfer's lift." This involves keeping one foot planted straight on the floor with your other foot going in the air as you reach down to pick up something. If you do not know what I am referring to, you can get a quick picture of this online. This is another great position that people prefer. According to the research, it also places less stress on the spine. Whether someone chooses this method or the prior method is up to them. I usually give people the option and let them decide which one feels best.

## Clinical Presentation

Typically, if a patient is suffering from a disc-related pathology, they will note several things. First off, they typically have increasing pain in the lower back when they bend forward, also known as flexion. Bending forward increases the pressure of the herniation because it causes the spine to round. Another position that increases pressure in this area is when a patient sits for a prolonged period of time. People tend to round their spines, thus increasing the pressure and pain in the affected areas.

A lot of the time, a person with a disc herniation will avoid these two positions. However, there is one position they may subconsciously find themselves in, and that position is extension. Extension is commonly known as bending backwards. If a patient has a true disc herniation that is pressing towards the back of the spine, going into spinal extension will give them relief because it causes the disc to go back into place.

If a patient's disc is herniated towards the back and the side, they may become symptomatic in side bending as well. Typically, you can tell if a person is doing this because they do not walk upright. If you think that you are altering your posture based on your pain, you should look at yourself standing in front of a mirror and make some postural fixes so that you are in an upright posture.

Since there is an association between having a herniated disc and sciatica, it is not uncommon to experience pain in these positions AND to have sciatica nerve pain at the same time. It is another sign that sciatica is caused by a herniated disc because these positions are stressing the disc. It is common for people to experience increasing lower back pain and sciatica pain as they sit or bend forward. Now that you have an understanding of what happens to the spine in these two positions, you know why that is the case. Both of these positions cause the spine to round and go into flexion, which is a common position to reproduce these symptoms.

## Peripheralization vs. Centralization

There are two terms that are important to know if you simultaneously have a herniated disc and sciatica pain. The first term is peripheralization, which essentially means that pain is traveling further from the spine. An example of this would be a person with lower back pain that extends down their thigh and goes into the back of their calf. Peripheralization typically occurs in a person's lower extremity. An increase in this type of pain usually indicates that the condition is worsening. If I am working with a person in a clinical setting and their leg pain starts to get worse, I immediately stop the exercise because my goal is to never make a person feel worse.

Centralization is just the opposite: it refers to pain that begins to move towards the spine. An example is that the same patient as before begins to experience relief in their calf but still has pain in their thigh and lower back. Then, after further treatment, they experience relief in their thigh and just have pain in their lower back. Finally, they begin to have relief in their lower back and the pain goes away completely. This is indicative of improvement because the nerve root is having pressure relieved from it.

I will go over a basic treatment in the next section. It is very important that you take note of what happens to your symptoms when you do it. If the symptoms begin to peripheralize, you should back off because you don't want to make your condition worse. If your symptoms begin to centralize, however, you know that things are starting to improve. One side note about centralization: sometimes symptoms will centralize, causing the sciatica to improve, BUT the lower back pain to worsen. Do not be alarmed by this. It is normal, but you should still progress slowly and gently through the exercises.

## Tests for Herniated Disc

Clinicians typically do the two tests that I went over earlier for sciatica to confirm a disc herniation. The slump test and straight leg raise test are both clinically proven to reproduce pain if a person is suffering from this condition. I personally use these two in the clinic because disc herniations and sciatica go hand in hand. If necessary, like before, it's beneficial to have findings followed up with imaging to confirm. These tests are performed in combination with a person's clinical presentation of having pain with motions that involve flexion. There are other tests out there that people like to include for disc herniations; however, these two are validated in the research community and I have personally had a lot of success with them.

## McKenzie Extension Exercise for Disc Herniation

If you know you have a disc herniation, there is an important exercise you should perform, known as the McKenzie exercise. This exercise is performed by placing the spine into extension, which in theory allows the disc to move back into place. Any time a patient comes to therapy with a herniated disc, this is the first exercise they must learn to do because it helps reverse the compressive load they have already put on the disc. The idea behind these exercises is that since you are reversing the motion of the spine that causes pain, over time it can cause the disc to take pressure off of the nerve. By going into extension, it is also hypothesized that the force causes the disc to go back into place. I have a supplemental video on my YouTube channel titled, "Low Back Herniated Disc Exercises – McKenzie Exercises for Lumbar Bulging Disc," if you would like a visual aid.

1. To begin, lie prone on your stomach in a straight line with a pillow under your chest. Try to maintain this position for 5-10 minutes. If you

experience relief with this position, then progress. If it is already difficult, continue lying in this position.

2. To progress from here, place your elbows under your shoulders and press up onto your elbows. Press up for a count of one and then go back down. Perform 10 repetitions.

3. For the next progression, place your hands under your shoulders now and press up with your hands. Only press up to where you can tolerate and then lower yourself back down. It's important that your hips maintain contact with the surface you are pressing up from. Perform 10 repetitions.

4. The next step is just like the prior one except that now you are pressing up until your arms are completely straight while maintaining contact with your hips. It is common that people shrug their shoulders up towards their ears when performing this. Therefore, it is important to keep your shoulder blades down and relaxed. Perform 10 repetitions.

5. The final position is pressing up until your elbows are completely straight, as before. However, this time you do a big exhale when you are in the press up position.

The primary goal with this exercise is that the pain will begin to centralize and then go away. I'll give you a typical presentation of a patient who has symptoms that are centralizing. If they come in with pain radiating from the lower back, down the back of their thigh, and into their calf, they may initially experience decreased pain in their calf. As they perform more of these exercises, the pain may then disappear from their thigh and only be present in their lower back. Finally, the pain may only be present in their lower back and then disappear completely. This ideal scenario is the goal of this exercise progression. One thing to note is that this exercise can be varied to focus more on one side of the spine compared to the other. For example, if you have a left-side disc herniation, you can shift your lower half to the left and then perform the progression outlined before. I suggest to people that they play around with what feels the best and what gives them the most relief.

**Standing Back Extension**

There may be times when people cannot lie down on the floor or a surface when they are experiencing their symptoms. If that is the case, they can still do a variation of the McKenzie extension exercise while standing. Although it is not as effective, in my opinion, it can still provide relief because it places the spine in extension.

1. Begin by standing up straight, push your hips forward, and bend backwards like you are trying to look at the ceiling. Perform 10 repetitions.

2. To progress this exercise, place both hands on your lower back and push your hips forward. Perform 10 repetitions.

3. Finally, if you would like to add some further extension, do a big exhale while pushing your hips forward. Perform 10 repetitions.

When you place both hands on your lower back, you add some overpressure that allows the spine to go into further extension. Adding that exhalation provides additional overpressure. Like before, you want to be cognizant of your symptoms and progress accordingly.

# CORE STRENGTH

One area that is continually harped on is core strength. Your core is extremely important when it comes to maintaining a stable and strong spine. Think of the core as a person's anatomical belt that supports them throughout movements. You may have seen people wear weightlifting belts in the gym. Their goal is to provide external support. A clinician named Stuart McGill is considered the lower back pain guru. He has done extensive research on core strength. He has determined that by training the core with isometric exercises, you can increase the core's stiffness and rigidity. When someone has a rigid and a stiff spine, it minimizes micromovements at the joints in the spine and prevents pain. Even if their sciatica pain is not directly caused by a disc herniation, it is still essential that they learn this to prevent further injury.

Isometric exercises are exercises that are done in static positions. A good example of an isometric core exercise is the plank. Isometric exercises differ from isotonic exercises in that the length of the muscle is changing with movement. A common example of an isotonic core exercise is the abdominal crunch. Now, I am not saying that you should avoid all isotonic exercises. However, I am saying that from a rehabilitation standpoint it is essential to include isometric core exercises in the recovery process. Therefore, I want to go over some plank variations that have been effective during my treatment of people with lower back pain.

Before I introduce these exercises, I want you to think of the core as a house that has 4 sides. If one side is weak, the house is not stable and might collapse. This same principle applies to the core, so it is important to be strong on all sides. Therefore, I incorporate core exercises that focus on the front of the core, the sides of the core, and the back of the core.

I also want to go into abdominal bracing briefly. This is when we tighten all of our core muscles simultaneously to protect the spine. Imagine that someone is about to punch you right in the stomach. You will tighten your stomach in anticipation. When I am teaching people these exercises, I always emphasize that they are bracing their core effectively. Initially, it may be difficult, but over time, as they learn this method, they find it becomes easier. When a person performs this abdominal bracing, it allows the protective musculature around the spine to tighten and further prevent movement. That is why it is essential to learn and develop during the rehabilitation process.

**Front Plank**

The front plank is an essential isometric core exercise that strengthens the front of your core. As it is commonly done incorrectly, I always go over how to properly perform a plank when treating a new patient.

1.  Begin on the floor on your hands and knees. Lower yourself to the floor onto your forearms with your elbows directly under your shoulders.

2. Contract your glutes in this position and perform abdominal bracing. If this is already a difficult position for you, hold this for up to 30 seconds. Work up to 4 sets.

3. Make sure you keep your spine all in alignment and keep your shoulders relaxed to prevent shrugging your shoulders up to your ears.

4. Be mindful not to allow your hips to sink down to the floor as well.

5. If you need to progress further, instead of having your knees come in contact with the ground, have your toes in contact with the ground instead.

6. The exercise can also be progressed by raising one foot off the ground to reduce the points of contact. This encourages additional stabilization at the core musculature to prevent the body from rotating.

It is important to make sure the spine stays in perfect alignment, regardless of what variation is being performed. I usually suggest to people that they watch themselves in a mirror or have somebody watch them. Also, maintaining the core and glute contraction throughout the movement is very important to provide a stable core. Neglecting these steps leads to the exercise not being performed properly and the core not being trained effectively. Finally, it's important to not allow the head to fall towards the ground when performing this exercise to prevent straining the neck.

**Side Plank**

The side plank is also a very essential isometric core exercise because it focuses more on your obliques. Just like the front plank, however, it is commonly done incorrectly. When done correctly, it will effectively strengthen the sides of your core.

1. To work your right obliques, begin by lying on the floor on your right side with your right elbow directly under your shoulder.

2. Perform abdominal bracing and make contact with the floor with your right knee and right forearm simultaneously. Contract your right glute in this position. If this is already a difficult position for you, hold this for up to 30 seconds. Work up to 4 sets and then repeat on the left side.

3. Make sure you keep your spine in alignment and that your right shoulder is related to prevent shrugging your shoulders up to your ears.

4. Be mindful not to allow your hips to sink down to the floor as well.

5. If you need to progress further, instead of having your knee come in contact with the ground, have your feet in contact with the ground.

6. Finally, the exercise may be progressed even further by raising the upper leg off the ground to reduce points of contact.

Sometimes people do this exercise with their feet stacked on top of each other, but I believe this places unnecessary strain on the ankles. Therefore, if you are doing a right side plank, I typically tell people to have both feet resting on the floor with their left foot placed in front of their right. This is repeated vice versa on the other side. I usually let people choose depending on what they are feeling.

**The Bird Dog Exercise**

The last exercise I really like to introduce to people to help with their core is known as the "bird dog" exercise. It is called this because you begin on all fours, hence the "dog," and then you raise your arms and legs, which resembles a "bird." Like the prior exercises, you may have seen other people do these, but not everybody performs them correctly. This is an essential stabilization exercise for the core because it is a very uncommon position that we are not naturally in. When done correctly, it is effectively strengthening the front of a person's core and the back.

1. To begin, go into the all fours position.
2. Perform abdominal bracing and straighten out your right leg as if you are trying to kick somebody behind you. Hold this position for 5-10 seconds and bring your leg back in. Then perform on the other side. Work up to 20 repetitions.
3. Be sure to maintain a straight line with your spine and do not allow your head to sink to the floor.
4. Make sure your shoulders remain relaxed and prevent them from shrugging up to your head.
5. To further advance this exercise, kick out your right leg and extend your left arm simultaneously. Then perform on the other side.

When people initially perform this exercise, they have a difficult time not falling over. That is why I always instruct them to straighten their legs first and then advance to the simultaneous leg and arm combination. A common mistake when people perform this exercise is that they raise their arms and legs too high. This will create hyperextension at the spine and can lead to pain. I always tell people to imagine that their body is a straight line and that their arms and legs are an extension of the spine. Keeping everything in line will work the appropriate muscles and should not increase symptoms.

# CLOSING THOUGHTS

I hope that by reading this guide and performing the exercises, you no longer feel helpless and lost in this entire process. If you are suffering from sciatica, it can be easy to feel discouraged and doomed. This can be a horrible condition that I have firsthand seen sideline people for a long period of time. If you have the right guidance and are incorporating up-to-date treatments, then relief can absolutely be experienced without surgery. In many cases, I have seen people become pain-free and get back to their daily activities without having to think about pain anymore. As a physical therapist, I really want to make sure that people can become independent when dealing with their ailments. People can accomplish this goal if they truly put in the work and listen to those that have the experience and knowledge. I hope that you find the information in this guide helpful because my goal is to help those suffering from sciatica nerve pain. I want to help people get back to living their lives pain-free because that is what I love doing day in and day out. One thing I will add is that if you use these treatments and start to feel better, just remember to keep up with the exercises and stretches to prevent the pain from coming back. A common theme in the physical therapy world is that once people get relief, they start to slack off with their exercises. Although not all the time, sometimes people start back at square one if they re-injure themselves. I hope that you have enjoyed what I had to say and I want to thank you for listening to me on this subject.

# REFERENCES

Boote J, Newsome R, Reddington M, Cole A, Dimairo M. Physiotherapy for Patients with Sciatica Awaiting Lumbar Micro-discectomy Surgery: A Nested, Qualitative Study of Patients' Views and Experiences. Physiother Res Int. 2016;22(3):e1665.

Brinjikji W, Luetmer PH, Comstock B, et al. Systematic Literature Review of Imaging Features of Spinal Degeneration in Asymptomatic Populations. *AJNR Am J Neuroradiol.* 2014;36(4):811-6.

Dutton, M. (2012). Orthopaedic Examination, Evaluation, and Intervention. New York: McGraw Hill Medical.

Jeong UC, Kim CY, Park YH, Hwang-Bo G, Nam CW. The Effects of Self-Mobilization Techniques for the Sciatic Nerves on Physical Functions and Health of Low Back Pain Patients With Lower Limb Radiating Pain. *J Phys Ther Sci.* 2016;28(1):46-50.

Kauppila LI, McAlindon T, Evans S, Wilson PW, Kiel D, Felson DT. Disc Degeneration/Back Pain and Calcification of the Abdominal Aorta. A 25-Year Follow-Up Study in Framingham. Spine (Phila Pa 1976). 1997;22:1642-1647, discussion 1648-9. 47.

Koes BW, van Tulder MW, Peul WC. Diagnosis and Treatment of Sciatica. *BMJ.* 2007;334(7607):1313-7.

Xiang A, Xu M, Liang Y, Wei J, Liu S. Immediate Relief of Herniated Lumbar Disc-Related Sciatica by Ankle Acupuncture: A Study Protocol for a Randomized Controlled Clinical Trial. *Medicine (Baltimore)*. 2017;96(51):e9191.

Wang D, Nasto LA, Roughley P, et al. Spine Degeneration in a Murine Model of Chronic Human Tobacco Smokers. Osteoarthritis Cartilage. 2012;20(8):896-905. 50.

# ABOUT THE AUTHOR

Nicholas Gallo is a board-certified doctor of physical therapy. He has helped countless patients in his career and continues to practice physical therapy on a full-time basis. He is also a cofounder of *Physical Therapy 101*.

# ADDITIONAL RESOURCES

For more information, visit my website at www.physicaltherapy101.net. Here we have resources on various pathologies. This website is continuously updated to provide up to date treatment and is a great resource for practitioners, patients, and prospective Physical Therapists.

Subscribe to my YouTube channel https://www.youtube.com/c/PhysicalTherapy101.

Here we produce free treatment videos for patients and healthcare providers. This is also a great visual aid for treatments described above.

I have other publications that you may also find interesting:

Posture Pain:  Key Strategies to Stay Pain Free at Your Desk and in Life – I discuss the optimal computer station setup to maintaining ideal posture, exercises to perform to reduce pain, and ways to implement these strategies in other scenarios.

Getting Into Physical Therapy School: 10 Essential Things You Must Do - If you are interested in a career in Physical Therapy this is the guide for you.  I go in depth on key strategies on how to get accepted into a Physical Therapy program. These strategies will strengthen your application and separate you from the competition.

Proper Bench Press Form: The Beginner's Guide to Warm-Up, Technique, and Injury Prevention - If you are a beginner to bench pressing or you are experienced but want to incorporate some injury prevention this is for you. You will learn how to warm up properly, ideal technique, and proven exercises to help with injury prevention.

P.S. If you have enjoyed this book and found it resourceful, please leave a helpful review on Amazon.

Lightning Source UK Ltd.
Milton Keynes UK
UKHW011836151219
355431UK00027B/133/P

9 781794 560024